Make Your Own Infused Water

The Healthy and Fun Way to Stay Hydrated

RON KNESS

ISBN-13: 978-1974059911
ISBN-10: 197405991X

Contents

Disclaimer

This publication is for informational purposes only and is not intended as medical advice. Medical advice should always be obtained from a qualified medical professional for any health conditions or symptoms associated with them.

Every possible effort has been made in preparing and researching this material. We make no warranties with respect to the accuracy, applicability of its contents or any omissions.

See your healthcare professional before starting any diet, health or exercise program!

Introduction

Infused water is the process of adding fruits, vegetables, and herbs to your water, then

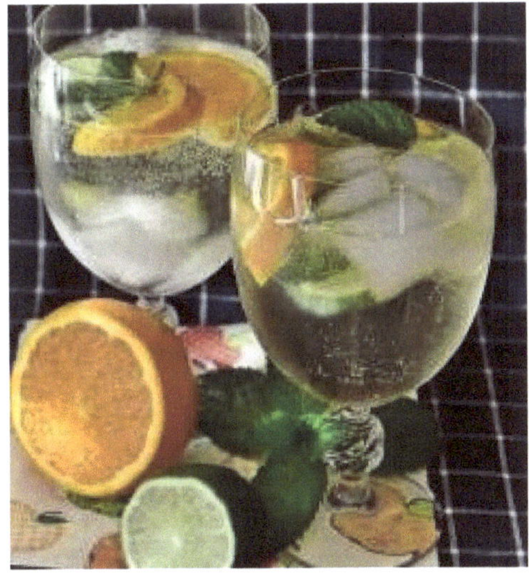

letting these ingredients flavor the water. In addition to providing a delicious flavor with a wide range of combination options, you also get some of the nutrients from the produce and herbs, which further improves how healthy your water is. Infused water is easy to do, but there are a few things you should know first. Here are some things to keep in mind when you are making your infused water.

Types of Water to Use

The first thing you should know about making infused water is that filtered water is always better. Filtered water is cleaner, so this is really going to improve the overall quality and flavor of your infused water.

Since not everyone has access to enough filtered water to fill **infused water pitchers** (http://amzn.to/2uKMNjA) every time, tap water is okay when necessary, but do try to get filtered water if at all possible.

When choosing your water, you should only use room temperature or cold water. Avoid warm or hot water, since it can cause the produce to fall apart at a rapid rate, which reduces how many nutrients are going to end up in your water.

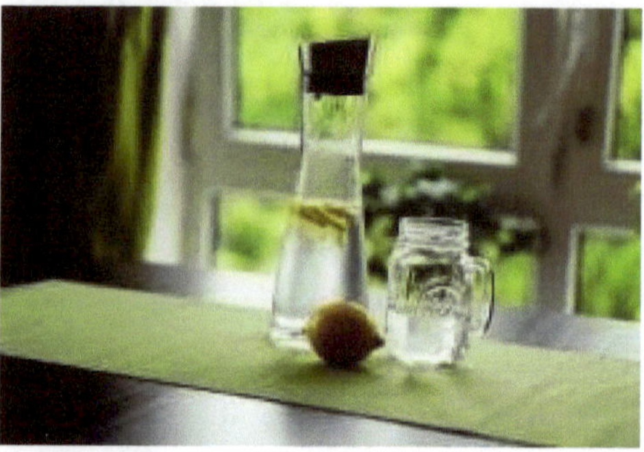

Choose Organic When Possible

If at all possible, try to select organic fruits and vegetables. These can often be found in the produce of your supermarket, but a better option might be to get them from a weekly CSA, farmer's market, or contacting local farmers directly. This allows you to get fresh fruits and veggies that you know were grown locally without added fertilizers and other chemicals. Organic produce does tend to provide a better flavor for infused water. However, the most important part is having healthy water with your favorite fruits and veggies, so if you can't use organic, don't worry too much about it!

How to Prep the Ingredients

After you select the ingredients you want to use for your infused water, you will then need to prep them before putting them into the pitcher. You should always rinse the fruits and vegetables to make sure no chemicals are left on them. Even if you bought them organic, it is still a good idea to rinse them and make sure they are clean. If you are using herbs, you want to crush them with a **muddler** (http://amzn.to/2vRwzVX) since this will help to release the oils.

The exception is when the herb is leafy, such as with mint or basil.

Most fruits and vegetables need to be cut at least in half before being put in the pitcher so that they can release their flavors. Hard fruits and vegetables like cucumber and apples need to be cut into thin slices since they can take longer to release flavor to the water. With berries and citrus fruit, they are softer, so just cutting them in half or quarters should be fine.

What to Make Your Infused Water In

By this point, you are ready to start putting your infused water together. Before you add in the water, make sure you have the right container. While you can technically use anything, a glass pitcher is usually recommended. However, regardless of which way you go, make sure it is BPA-free and food-safe.

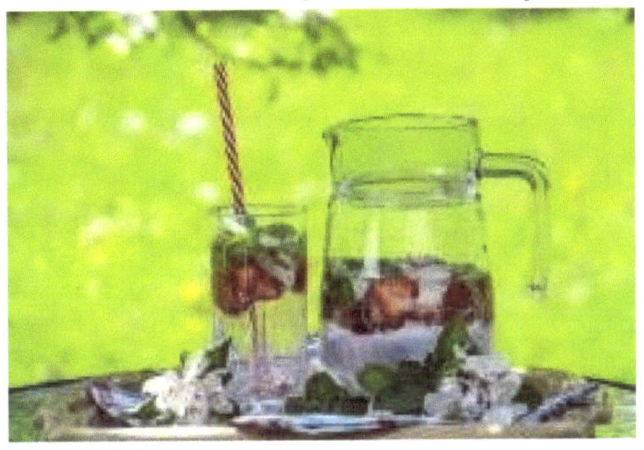

Many plastic pitchers are not ideal and won't keep the water fresh, but in the end it is really up to you.

There are also **pitchers** (http://amzn.to/2uKMNjA) and **bottles** (http://amzn.to/2uHfJL3) used especially for infusing. They typically have a long and narrow section in the middle where you put your herbs and fruit, with holes or slots so the flavor can be released. You can use these, but they aren't necessary.

How Long to Soak the Produce

When making infused water, you will add the produce and herbs first, then add your room temperature or cold water on top.

You then want to let the water infuse so that you can get good flavors and nutrients from the fruits and vegetables being used. If you are leaving it out on the counter, this is usually done in about 2 hours.

Otherwise, wait 4-6 hours if keeping it in the refrigerator for the infusing process. If you leave it overnight, it will be super flavorful.

When the Water Should Be Enjoyed

The ideal time to drink infused water is within 24-48 hours after the infusing process is complete. It is usually best to drink it the same day, but at least try to drink it within the first couple days. Waiting 3 days is okay, but don't leave it for longer than that.

Make sure you are not leaving the fruits and vegetables in the water for this long though. They should be removed and only the water should remain in the pitcher for this long. Citrus fruits will remain fresher for longer, while melons are going to get soft and mushy quickly.

Also keep in mind that if you drink the infused water the same day, you can usually refill it 2-3 times with the produce in the pitcher or cup and still get good flavor from it.

Why Everyone Should Drink Infused Water

As people turn away from the sugar-filled drinks aimed at both adults and children, people everywhere are beginning to look for alternatives to these overly sweet soft drinks. For some, juice can be extremely expensive, especially if they are looking for fresh juices that can take the place of soda and the high fructose corn syrup based juice boxes. One solution that could provide a refreshing taste and plenty of hydration, is infused water. If you continue reading, you can learn about some of the great reason why everyone should have a glass.

You Will Fight Oxidation

Oxidation in the human body can manifest in various ways, but the most common is usually age spots, which is a literal organic equivalent to rust. Infused water uses a lot of types of fruit that contain heavy doses of antioxidants. Beyond being very tasty and great for your general health, these antioxidants can help you to fight the effects of human oxidation, which causes aging and lots of other negative effects. Antioxidants can also fight the free radicals that can help to contribute to the conditions needed to make cancer a possible outcome.

It Can Prevent Kidney Stones

Kidney stones can be continuous problem for some people. If you discover that you have them, it could mean expensive medical treatments for days or even weeks. The more natural method of dealing with these irritating mineral deposits is to ingest generous amounts of fruit.

You can also prevent them by drinking infused water. This works because the acids contained in a large portion of fruit can prevent the formation of the stones, and keep you from ever having to deal with them at all.

You Will Get More Hydration

Drinking water should be a major portion of what people ingest in a day, but that isn't always the case. Depending on local culture, some people will lean more towards store bought and manufactured choices of hydration. Not only are these forms of hydration far less healthy, they are normally far less effective at delivering the appropriate amount of water that the body needs, because water is a basic need for the human body like oxygen. There is no complete substitute.

Drinking infused water will give you nutrients, and hydration that will help your body to feel more healthy and ready to perform the complex tasks that it needs to function properly.

5 Simple Tricks to Help You Drink More Water Every Day

Did you know that simply drinking more water can repel and even treat Alzheimer's disease? Water flushes your system, and regulates a healthy digestive tract. Water promotes heart health and a strong circulatory system. Your body is roughly 60% water, and uses up some of your water supply each day. That water has to be replaced.

The problem is, you probably are not drinking enough. The average adult needs to drink at least 1 gallon of water each and every day for optimal health. Practice the following 5 simple tricks to help you drink more water on a daily basis, and your health will see a positive boost.

1 - Make a goal and stick to it – Human beings are great goal setters and achievers. If you just think about drinking more water in the back of your mind, you may be successful, or you may not. However, if you write down a specific goal for daily water consumption you program the habit-forming part of your brain to increase your water intake.

2 - Plan for it – Keep gallons or liters of fresh water on hand at all times. Store some in your refrigerator for a cool and refreshing zero calorie treat that also helps fight hunger pangs. Keep bottled water at your job, in your vehicle, at home and in your backpack when you are on the go. The more water available, the more likely you are to drink this healthy beverage rather than an unhealthy, sugar-filled and processed alternative.

3 - Buy a really nice water bottle — Don't just head to your local $1 store for this purchase. Find a good-looking, functional, BPA-free water bottle you really like. If you are proud to display your new healthy habit, you are much more likely to stick to it.

4 - There's an app for that — It seems there is an application for just about anything. This includes apps like Daily Water, iDrated, Waterlogged and Eight Glasses a Day. They make it easy to track your water consumption on a daily basis, and range from free to just $.99 per download.

5 - Add healthy natural flavor — Why not pop some blueberries, cucumbers, strawberries, limes or orange slices into your water? When you are done drinking, you enjoy a healthy fruit or vegetable snack. You can also add your favorite herbs for a wonderful aroma while you hydrate. yourself naturally.

6 - Use mineral water - For a different liquid than just plain water, try making your infusion with mineral water. Use unflavored or choose from flavored water. Boost up the flavor by adding your own fruits, herbs and vegetables.

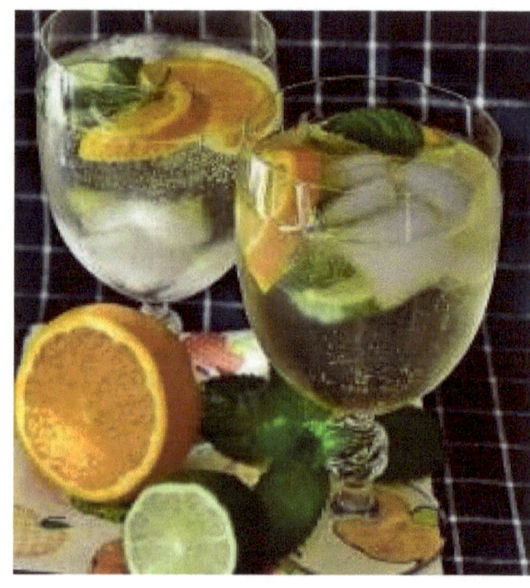

The 3-Step Process to Making Infused Water

If you've been looking for a healthy drink that you can have anytime of the day that makes you feel healthy and refreshed, then infused water is probably a great option for you. This great drink is the choice of many healthy people who want to be able to enjoy a glass of something that will give them real vitamins and minerals, while giving them the hydration their body craves, but if you're new to this concept, you might want to know a few things about how it's done, so this article will be showing you how to make your own infused water.

Get A Good Container

When you want to make some infused water, the first thing that you really need to have is a good sealable container. If you have large jars that you would like to use or anything of that sort, there should be tight fitting lids that go on them. For larger quantities, a glass pitcher works great, but make sure it is glass and not plastic.

Choose Your Ingredients

The secret to a great infused water recipe is the freshest ingredients that you can get your hands on. Typically, you will want them to be organic so they have the full amount of nutrients and are unlikely to contain any kind of pesticides.

You can use herbs like mint, rosemary, or thyme. You should also select what kinds of fruits or vegetables that you are going to be including in your recipe. This will form the flavor that you're hoping to achieve, or you can simply look up some recipes that have already been written. Some sample recipes to get you started are included in this book. It's important to be sure to exclude any pieces that show signs of rot or deterioration, because it could taint the batch.

Put Them In The Water And Wait

After you've selected your chosen mixture, place it in the water and close the lid. It will take some time for it to flavor the water in a way that will give it the properties that it should have. Generally, you will want it to sit for at least 3 hours, but some herbs might take a little longer.

It's definitely a good idea to wait as long as you can stand it, because the longer it sits, the more flavor and potency it will have. You might want to put it in the refrigerator so that it can stay fresh and cool. After it's done, you can enjoy a refreshing healthy drink!

Simple Infused Water Recipes to Start With

Infused water can be a really awesome and fun way to get a few nutrients. Another great thing about it, is that your body will love it because actual water is way more hydrating than any of the drinks that are marketed and being great for hydration.

One thing you might be wondering though, is how to get started with making infused water. Fortunately, you're about to begin reading about everything you'll need to know about making your very own batches of infused water.

What You'll Need

First of all, fill your container a little more than ¾ the way up with some filtered or tap water, and grab your favorite ingredients. Pitchers are also great for infused water if you want to make a larger batch.

Citrus and Mint

Here is a really great recipe that will refresh and cool you down. Find your favorite citrus fruit and cut it into fourths.

Slice each of the fourths into slices with peel that are about a centimeter wide and place them in the container filled with water. Grab a few pieces of freshly picked mint leaves, and you might even want them still on the entire shoot. Let the drink sit for at least 4 - 5 hours before drinking because mint will take some time to absorb completely. Ice can be optional.

Kiwi Blackberry

This is a great recipe full of powerful antioxidants. Peel 2 kiwis and slice them into coins that are about half a centimeter each. Place the kiwi slices into the water, then lightly agitate or lightly break apart some blackberries and drop them into the water. Be sure to let the mixture sit for a while until the water begins to take on some of the color of the berries. Once the water no longer gets any darker than it is ready.

Pineapple Cucumber

This drink can be great and helps you to get extra water off of your body. Slice the pineapple into about 3 - 4 rings that are about a centimeter wide, and then cut the rings in 8 sections. Cut the cucumber into coins that are about a half centimeter or less in thickness, and place all of it into the water. Let the water sit until it begins to color, or about 4 hours.

Simple Veggie and Fruit Infused Water Combinations

If you're familiar with infused water somewhat, you've likely seen quite a few combinations of fruit that you can use to create tasty and refreshing drinks for your own year-round enjoyment, but did you know that there are some recipes that can get you some of the amazing benefits of vegetables as well? Keep reading to get some amazing new recipes that use both vegetable and fruit combinations for some really great drinks.

Strawberry Lime Cucumber

Cucumber makes a great addition to almost any infused drink. Limes are an excellent source of vitamin C, and citric acids, which help to break down mineral deposits in the gallbladder. Take some strawberries and drop them into the water. They can be cut or whole. Then, cut the lime into coins. Make them thin and you can leave the skin on. After that is done, cut the cucumber into coins and

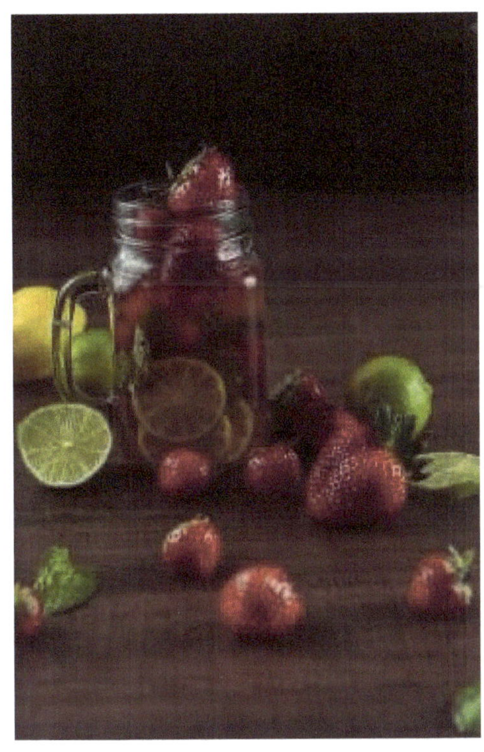

place all of the cut matter into the container. Let it sit for about 3 hours and you'll have a great healthy drink. It can also help you to lose weight.

Tomato Celery Basil

Here is a drink that has more fragrant flavor. The celery should be organic so that you don't ingest as many pesticides from your food. Cut a long stalk of celery into strips and place it into the water. Cut the tomato into 8 slices and put it into the container. Then, put in a shoot of basil and let it sit for 5 - 6 hours.

Celery is highly alkaline and will help to control stomach acids. Tomato is good at helping the body to control cholesterol.

Cucumber Lemon Watermelon

If you need serious vasodilation, watermelon is a good thing to put in your infused drinks. Lemons are high in vitamin C, so they can help you to strengthen your immune system.

To make this drink, cut the cucumber into coins and place them into the water. After this step is finished, cut the lemon into coins and drop it into the water. You can leave the rind on the watermelon of you like, but cut the watermelon into cubes or any other fun shapes.

Mint Cucumber Jalapeno

This one is pretty straight forward. Heavy dose of vitamin C, drop in mint, cut cucumber into coins and then make a slit into a single jalapeno. Let it sit for 3 hours and serve chilled.

Health Benefits of Lemon Water

One of the healthiest, easiest to make and best tasting infused water in my opinion is simple lemon water. When it comes to taking better care of yourself, you have probably heard of drinking more water as one of the best things you can do. However, it is also helpful to add something to the water, such as lemon juice or lemon slices. Take a look at these different health benefits of drinking lemon water.

It Cleanses Your System

One of the top benefits of lemon water is the fact that it can

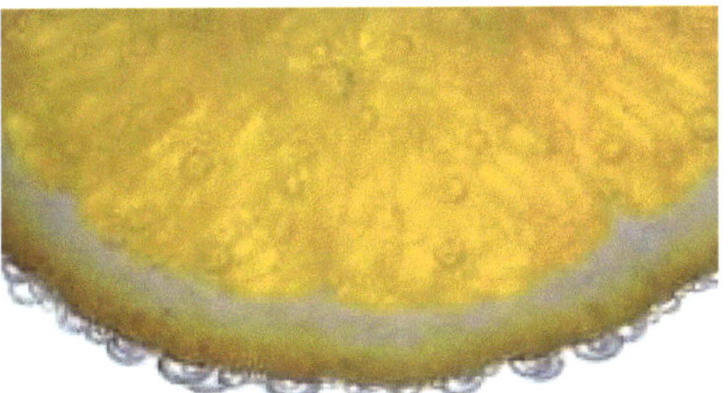

help to cleanse all those toxins out of your body. It is one of the easiest and most natural ways to detox your body. You also don't need to do an extreme detox just to cleanse your system. Having a tall glass of lemon water every day will really do wonders for your body. You can improve enzyme function and help to clean out your liver as well.

Lemon Water is Great For Your Skin

You can also get some excellent health benefits for your skin from the inside out by drinking more lemon water. When you drink water with some lemon slices or lemon juice in it, you get all that wonderful vitamin C into your body. This combined with better hydration from the water is going to clear up your skin and get rid of free radicals that often cause damage to your skin. The vitamin C in the lemons can also help to promote more collagen production.

It Helps You Lose Weight

If you are currently trying to lose weight and get healthy, lemon water is the perfect thing to start with. Not only are you getting water with vitamin C from the lemon, but you are adding to the flavor of your water. This can help to encourage you to drink more of the water each day, which as you know is important for weight loss. Lemon water can also help to boost your metabolism, especially if you drink warm lemon water in the morning before consuming anything else.

Vitamin C is Great For Your immune System

Speaking of the vitamin C in lemon water, you are also helping to give your immune system a nice boost. All of the nutrients in lemons are going to transfer to the water, so you get those nutrients for optimal health. Vitamin C is good for your immune system, helping you to avoid the cold, flu, and various other illnesses. Try one or two glasses of lemon water each day for general health.

Infused Water Recipes Featuring Tropical Fruit

Infused water is all the rage right now. If you are giving up soda because of some of the health hazards associated with it and are looking for a safe drink that not only hydrates you but has some health benefits, try these refreshing recipes. By now you've probably seen a few recipes that use herbs, spices, apples, berries, and other common fruit, but what about something a little more off the beaten path? Here are some great ways to use tropical fruit for your next fruit-infused water.

Pineapple Ginger

Here is a nice tropical drink that can help you to stay healthy as well. Take a pineapple and slice off 3 - 4 rings. Cut the pineapple rings into at least 8 pieces and drop it into the container of water. Skin and cut 2, one-inch pieces of ginger off of the root piece and put it into the mixture. Let it sit for about 3 hours with the lid on. You can keep it chilled by adding some ice cubes or placing it into the refrigerator. The water should take on a yellowish tint when it is ready. Serve in glasses.

Champagne Mango and Lime

The Champagne Mango is a wonderful fruit from near the equator. It is smaller than many other varieties and has a unique flavor. With skin on, cut the mango into thin slices and place it into the water. Cut the lime into smaller wedges by cutting it into fours, then cutting those in half.

Place them into the water and let it sit at room temperature for about 4 hours. Keep chilled directly following the infusion. You can also add some orange to get a more robust flavor.

Acai Pomegranate

Acai is a wonderful fruit that is very high in antioxidants and essential vitamins and minerals. It pairs very well with pomegranate which is also very good for the body, particularly when it comes to inflammation. Cut the acai in to fours and place it into the water.

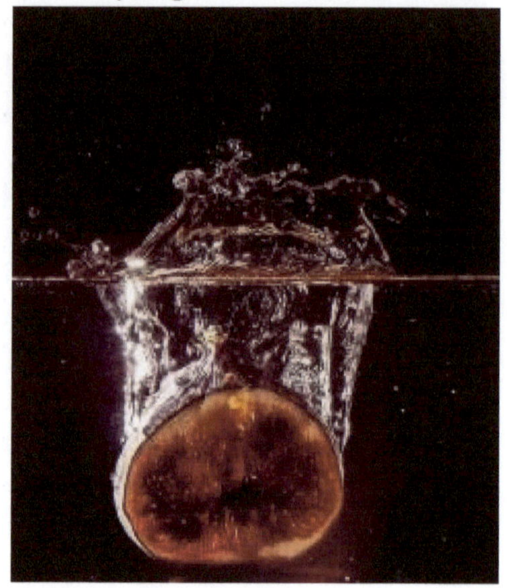

Then cut the pomegranate into smaller pieces like fours or whatever suits you best. Place it into the water and allow it to infuse for a minimum of 4 hours, but you may want to leave this mixture overnight for a better outcome.

Once it is finished, the water should have taken on a much darker appearance. If you like, you can choose to garnish the drink with mint or basil to give it some extra kick.

Fruit and Herb Infused Water for the Fall

When the fall season arrives, it is common to feel more festive and engaged in the holiday cheer. This season is full of great colors and flavors that can warm the chilliest of days. That is one reason why seasonal drinks are so popular, but have you ever come across any recipes for festive infused drinks? This chapter explores some ideas for festive fruit and herb infused drinks that you can enjoy in the fall.

Cranberries and Rosemary

This drink will be very reminiscent of great holiday dishes. Rosemary is also full of amazing essential oils that have their own benefits. It is also heavily anti-inflammatory. When you pick your piece of rosemary, be sure that it is very fresh. Place it in the water so it is completely covered. Add a handful of cranberries and let it sit overnight. The next day you'll have a great festive drink. You can also add basil for a richer more fragrant flavor.

Peppermint Strawberry

Who doesn't love candy canes? Some fresh peppermint with strawberry can put you in that holiday mood quickly, and the benefits of having peppermint can be far reaching, especially when it comes to its stomach soothing abilities.

It is also very handy at fighting various forms of gastrointestinal inflammation, which makes it a great treatment for Irritable Bowel Syndrome and other gastric inflammatory conditions.

Place a shot of peppermint into a large container. You can cut or leave the strawberries whole. Let it sit for at least 3 hours and serve.

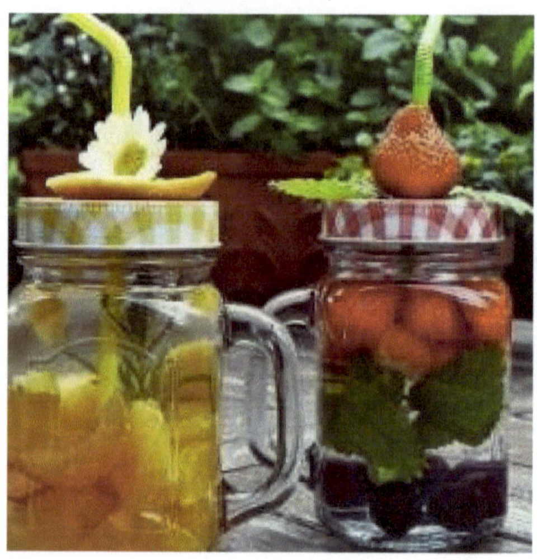

Cherry Mint

Cherries have a potent and tart taste. One amazing thing about cherries is that they are great in helping with inflammation of the joints. This makes them a good way to help with arthritis and other inflammatory disorders. The mint in the drink can also help with promoting digestion. Simply break off a fresh piece of mint and place it in the water. Place a handful of cherries in the water and let it sit overnight.

Seasonal Recipes

Apple Cinnamon

This simple apple cinnamon infused water recipe is easy to make, only uses a couple ingredients, and is perfect for the fall and winter season.

You can also mix it up by using some other seasonings with the same apples for a seasonal infused water. This recipe is great with a whole pitcher of infused water, or you can use a mason jar.

Ingredients:

- Red apples

- Cinnamon sticks

Directions:

1. Core and slice the apples thinly.

2. Place the apple slices and cinnamon stick in pitcher.

3. Add cold water.

4. Place in refrigerator for up to 24 hours.

Cranberry Orange

There are few things better than the combination between cranberry and orange. Both of these fruits are in season during the fall, and cranberry is often enjoyed during the holidays. This is a fruity and refreshing infused water to enjoy early in the morning or with your meals.

Ingredients:

- Cranberries

- Oranges

- Herbs (optional)

Directions:

1. Slice your cranberries in half to help release the juice.

2. Slice oranges thinly.

3. Add the cranberries and orange slices to a pitcher or infusing bottle.

4. Add in some herbs of your choice; mint and basil work well.

Fall Fruits

This is an infused water recipe with a lot of room for customizing. The basis of the recipe uses fruits that are in-season during the fall. This recipe is going to list a lot of fruits, but go ahead and use any of the ones listed that you want in this water.

Ingredients:

- Pears

- Apples

- Cranberries

- Tangerines

- Oranges

- Limes

Directions:

1. Cut fruit into small slices. Cut cranberries in half or use dried cranberries.

2. Add the fruit to the pitcher.

3. Cover the fruit with cold water and fill the pitcher to the top.

4. Add any herbs you like to increase flavor.

5. Place in the refrigerator for up to 48 hours.

Green Apple and Herbs

This is an excellent way to create your own fall fruit-infused water without worrying too much about what goes in it. You want to start with some juicy, tarty green apples since they are in-season, then add herbs or berries of your choosing. Rosemary is listed, but you can add mint, basil, or cilantro if you prefer.

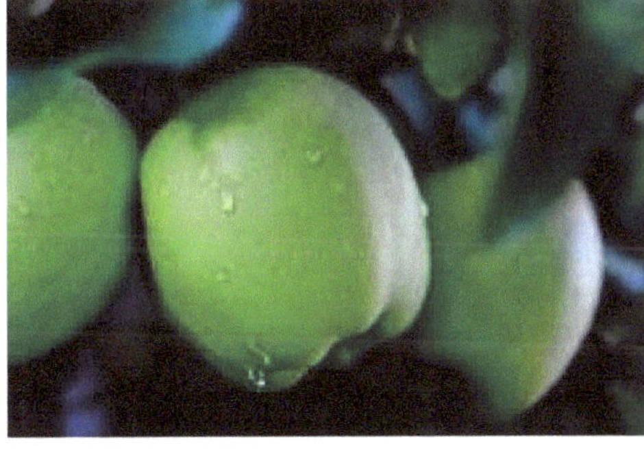

Ingredients:

- Green apples

- Berries (recommended: strawberries, cranberries, raspberries)

- Herbs (recommended: rosemary, basil, mint)

Directions:

1. Slice the apple thinly and add to the pitcher.

2. Add your chosen berries and herbs.

3. Fill the pitcher or cup with cold, distilled water.

4. Store for 24-48 hours.

Lime Pomegranate

Pomegranates are in season during the fall and winter season. These are brightly-colored fruits that offer a unique flavor and a lot of sweetness to your water. Combine it with lime for a delicious and refreshing water.

Ingredients:

- Pomegranate seeds

- Limes

Directions:

1. Scoop pomegranate seeds from your pomegranate fruit.

2. Muddle the seeds, add to the pitcher or cup.

3. Place slices of lime on top of the seeds.

4. Fill with cold, distilled water and handful of ice cubes.

Infused Water Recipes for Your Cocktails

The secret to any truly great mixed drink is almost always due to the kind of thing that you're mixing with your alcohol of choice. It can be hard to make a healthy choice though when you're looking for this magical additive.

Some people might want to have something that's a lot lower in sugar than most traditional mixers, so you might have your work cut out for you, but if you were to use infused water for your mixer, you could have the health benefits of the infusion and the flavor.

Blackberry Sage Gin

Fill a large jar a bit more than half way. Take some sage shoots and place them in the water. Be sure the sage is completely submerged. After that, add some blackberries to the mixture and let it sit in a cool environment for about 3 hours or more.

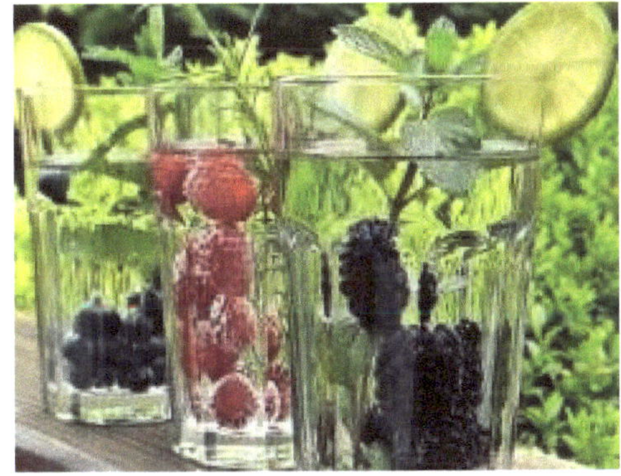

You'll know it's essentially finished once you see color in the water. Once it's finished, you can fill a glass about ⅔ the way full and add one shot of your favorite gin. This water also works great with other types of liquor.

Strawberry Lemon Rose Vodka

For this elegant and refreshing drink, you will want to gather a small handful of rose petals, then slice a lemon into wedges. You can either leave the strawberries as is, or you can cut them in half. Once everything is prepped, place them in the water and let it sit for at least 4 hours, but it would be even better if you let it sit overnight.

When you come to see it the next day it should have a beautiful color to the water. You can leave the plant material in, or strain it out. Fill your glass ⅔ the way full and add a shot of your favorite vodka, and you will have a memorable and delicious beverage.

Apple Cinnamon Rum

This drink could be considered sort of festive. Cut about 2 apples into very thin slices and place it into the water. Sprinkle in some cinnamon and stir. Let it sit for about 4 hours.

Once your infused apple drink is ready, pour some into a cup about ⅔ the way and add a shot of your favorite rum. If you want to add a little more kick to the mix, you can cut up a lime very thin and place that in with the apples.

Low-Carb Friendly Infused Water Ideas

If you've been trying to cut back on the carbs, and it's essential that you be as extremely strict with your intake, it can be very difficult to stick to a low carb program. This is because nearly everything that is available to drink contains some measure of carbs, or a ridiculous amount of sugar.

One great way to get yourself a refreshing drink would be to try and make some infused water. Infused water can easily be low in carbs and will give you the refreshing flavor and nutrients that your body needs.

Peach Cantaloupe

This great recipe is full of excellent and important vitamins and minerals. Cantaloupe is a good source of omega 3 fatty acids and other vitamins. 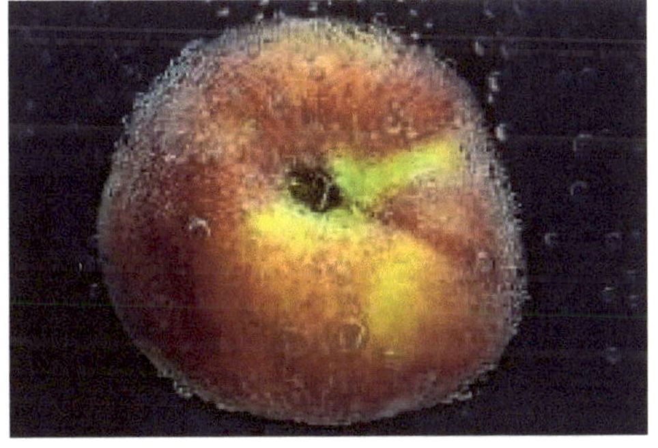 Peaches are a great source of many of the important minerals like phosphorus and manganese. Simply cut a peach into thin slices and place it in the water with some small cantaloupe cubes.

Let it sit for about 3 hours or until the water takes on a golden color. Enjoy it with ice if you want it chilled.

Peach is on the lower end of the carb spectrum, but cantaloupe can be too high for extremely low-carb diets. Therefore, depending on how much you are reducing your carbs, you might want to use twice as much peach as cantaloupe.

Strawberry Watermelon

Strawberries and watermelons are both lower in carbs than fruit like apples. Watermelon contains important nutrients that help with arterial health. Cut your watermelon into cubes. You can either leave the strawberries whole or cut them in half.

Place the fruit in the water and let it sit for at least 3 hours, but you may want to wait to try this mix until the following day when the water will be fully infused with amazing properties! A dash of mint is always welcome with watermelon if you want to kick things up a notch.

Watermelon Cucumber Mint

Mint is a great herb to put with watermelon because it is very refreshing to the mouth and stomach. Cucumber is great for stimulating the elimination of excess water from the body.

When you put these ingredients together, you end up with a tasty and refreshing drink with great perks. Cube some watermelon, cut cucumber into coins, and throw in a shoot of mint. Let it sit for at least 3 hours.

Strawberry Ginger

This one is pretty simple. It has antibacterial properties as well. Take a handful of strawberries and toss them into a

container with two, 1-inch long pieces of ginger. Let it sit overnight and you will have a great low carb drink that can help you keep your stomach healthy.

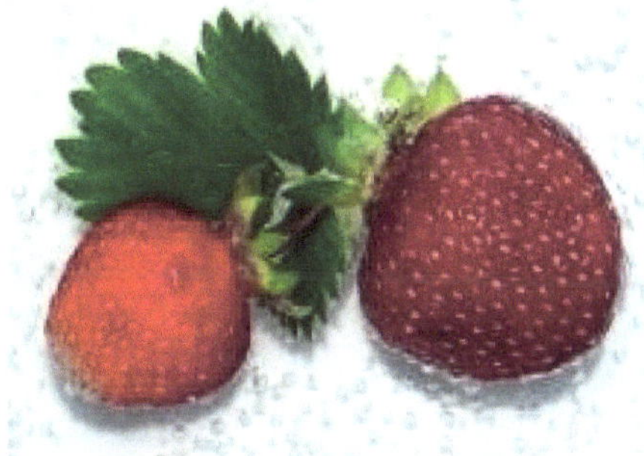

Herb-Infused Detox Water Recipes

Herbs are well known for their ability to medicate and heal the human body. For thousands of years, humans have used these simple plants to increase their quality of life, and to treat various diseases, and many of them happen to have a pleasing flavor!

Infused water has made a big comeback as a way to deliver healthy properties found in herbs. As you continue reading, you will find that this chapter contains a short list of recipes for helpful herb infused detox recipes.

Watermelon Basil

Basil is a powerful antioxidant and antimicrobial herb. This makes it a great herb for the infusion process. Be sure to grab a freshly picked piece of basil for this drink. Place the basil pieces in the water and add your watermelon chunks.

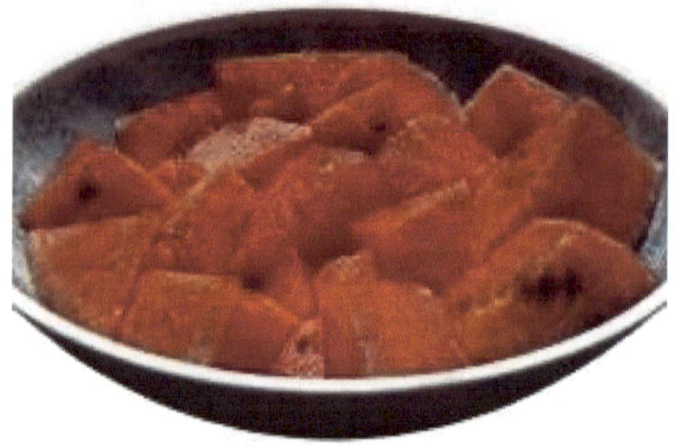

Let it sit overnight for the best results. Once it's ready, you can put it into a glass for a healthy drink.

Mint Cucumber

Mint has long been used to treat stomach issues and respiratory problems. It can also help you to fight off inflammation.

Cucumber is great at reducing water by promoting proper elimination.

Be sure that you have the very freshest mint that you can get your hands on.

Place the mint and cucumber into the water after you've cut the cucumber into coins about ¼ of a centimeter. Let it sit for about 3 hours and it should be ready to drink.

Lavender Blueberry

Lavender is heavily associated with skin health and sleep promotion. It is famous for helping people to cure forms of psoriasis. Blueberries are an excellent source of antioxidants. These berries are famous for fighting aging, and 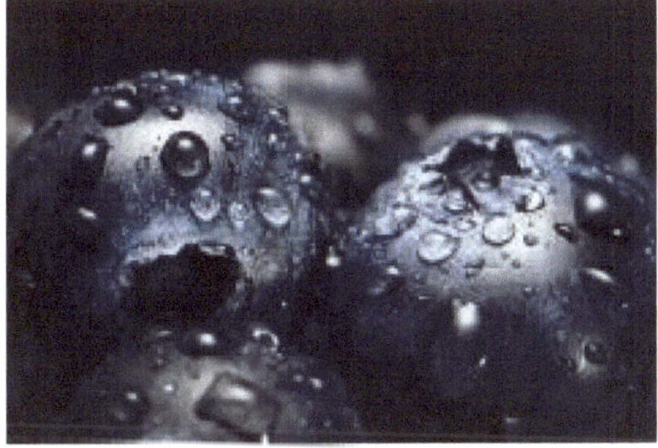 cancer. Place a handful of blueberries into the water with some freshly picked Lavender.

Let it sit for an entire night for the best results. Drink it with some ice or keep it chilled in the refrigerator for healthier skin and better sleep!

Sage Blackberry

Sage is well known for its positive effects on digestion and appetite, as well as depression. It quickly soothes the stomach to reduce bloating and is commonly used as a remedy for diarrhea. Blackberries are antioxidant and help to combat free radicals that cause cellular anomalies that led to cancer.

Let it sit in the water overnight for best results. When it is ready it should take on a darker color. Serve it up with or without ice for a powerful and useful remedy.

How to Make Fruit-Infused Ice Cubes

Infused water is a great way to get fast healthy hydration with just a bit of vitamins and minerals. Moms who want to keep healthy drinks in the home for their kids have turned to infused water as a substitute for the store-bought drinks, but what else can you do with infused water?

Ice cubes made of infused water can add a fun, flavorful edge to your favorite drinks, so this chapter will be sharing just a few ways to make fruit infused ice cubes.

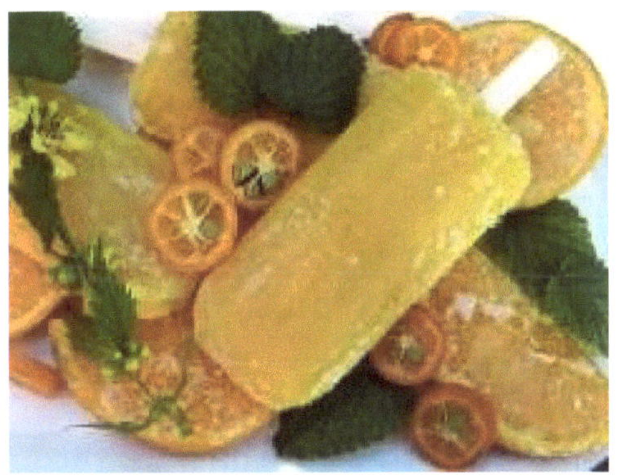

What You Will Need

The first thing you always need to make infused water is a sealable container, like a very large sealing jar. You will need some fresh fruits, herbs, and spices. Select only the freshest ingredients. After that, find some ice cube trays.

Trays can come in different sizes and shapes, so you can feel free to get imaginative or find one that best suits your purposes.

Some trays will offer shapes other than cubes, like the kind that have 10 - 12, 4 to 5-inch ice sticks.

Mint Sage Cubes

These cubes can add some soothing and unique flavor to your drinks. Take some fresh sage and mint and submerge in a water container. Let it sit for at least 3 - 4 hours.

Once it's ready, pour it into the ice tray. Try to make sure that you get a small amount of mint in each for looks and additional flavor as it melts. Place in the freezer until frozen and you'll have something that people remember for a long time with their drinks.

Cranberry Watermelon Sticks

If you can find these kinds of trays, then you'll have some really cool flavorful ice for some drinks. Place some cubed watermelon into the water along with some cranberries. Berry drinks typically take a bit longer to infuse, so it might be a good idea to leave this one overnight to gain its full flavor.

Once it's ready, you can pour the mix into the long cube tray. Once frozen, you'll have long ice pieces that can poke out of the drinks in an attractive way.

Blueberry Lavender

Place some lavender pieces in the water with some blueberries and let it sit overnight. Once the water is colored, place it in an ice cube tray and freeze with pieces in each cube. It makes for an attractive and flavorful presentation!

Final Thoughts

With soda – both diet and regular – falling out of favor with many people, infused water is a great alternative to stay hydrated. And there are so many combinations that keep it interesting and fun.

The recipes shared in this book are only the tip of the iceberg. Many more can be found searching the Internet, Pinterest or just let your imagination run wild!

If you don't have the time or desire to make your own infused water, you can buy it ready-made. Just be sure to read the nutrition label to ensure it does not have any added sugar or other unwanted ingredients.

Regardless of if you make your own or buy it already made, you owe it to yourself to not only enjoy the refreshing hydration infused water provides, but also the health benefits from the vitamins, minerals and other nutrients in it. Enjoy!

About the Author

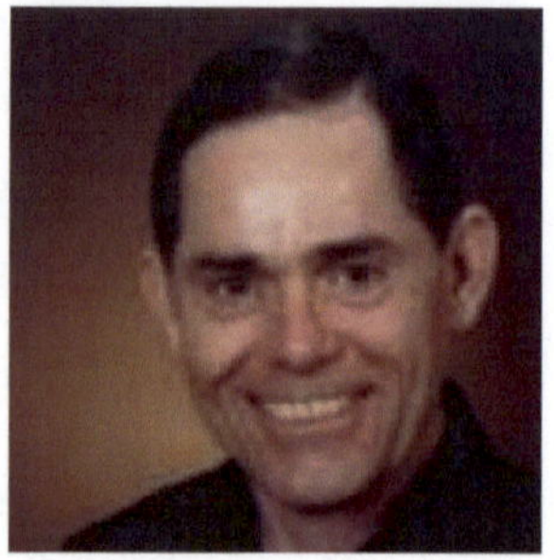

I have published over 170 books on Amazon for Kindle, CreateSpace and other publishing platforms.

While most of my books are on health and fitness in general, as I age (now 66) at the time of this writing) my topics of interest are geared toward aging baby boomers and older.

Besides my own writing, I also ghostwrite ebooks, books, reports, articles, blogs and do Kindle conversions for clients on a variety of topics.

Today my wife and I are retired from our careers and live in Gold Canyon, AZ. I now write as a retirement business where you'll find me happily sitting in my office typing away on my laptop as I work on my next book or ghostwriting project . . . that is if we are not traveling on a cruise ship - our new-found mode of travel.